MENTAL IMMUNITY

A GUIDE FOR EMOTIONAL RESILIENCE,
MASTERING EMOTIONS, AND MENTAL
TOUGHNESS

RICHARD NORMAN

CONTENTS

INTRODUCTION

We have all suffered some forms of conflict or abuse in our lives. But here's what I discovered: how we react to that abuse that will strengthen or weaken us. For example, everyone has dreams, right? But, how many of us have had a dream kicked to the curb? Can you remember what you wanted to be? Or do you have a dream right now tucked away in the back of your mind?

Have you ever been convinced to walk away from your dream by people who managed to throw enough self-doubt at you to win that war of attrition, the constant day in and day out negative input that pushes you to give up your dreams and conform to something you're not! "What are you nuts? You can't do that!" "Oh, there's another hair-brained scheme!" "Get Real! Go get a real job!" "Who do you think you are? You aren't something special; stick to the things you can handle." "What, are you stupid or something? Why do you think you can do that?" Lambasting you with negativity and giving you the message, " Who are you to become an author, or an inventor, or any number of other things your dreams may lead you to?" The litany goes on and on.

Often, the words that sting the most come from the people closest to us; I once heard that negative words were sixteen times more powerful than positive words, especially if they came from people you love. Unfortunately, many of us have heard similar comments from our own families. And remember that "family" is not just relatives but our closest circle of influence, the people that influence you the most in your life on a day-to-day basis.

We must learn how to reinforce our mental immune systems. As you are just opening up to re-affirming and re-discovering your dreams, it is important not to leave yourself open to Dream using attacks. Of course, when you are in the early creative process, you want to share that with the people closest to you, but too many times, you get shot down by those around you and can be stopped before you even begin. We already have to deal with our internal dream busters, voices from our past that can wreak havoc in our present.

It is amazing how many of us constantly go through life creating a speaking and thinking negative affirmations all day long to ourselves, "I always do that, I'm so stupid, etc." causing our ill emotional and mental states, yet we often have such an aversion to the idea that positive affirmations will have the same impact (but in the desired direction.) Pessimism and negativity are a much more accepted form of self-talk. However, recognizing it can be difficult. Sometimes it takes the form of a mental pause where suddenly you start to doubt yourself, and your dream seems to waver. Perhaps you start to wonder about your ability.

Become aware of this and catch it at that moment, realize that it is a trigger. Learn to recognize when you are being "infected" by those around you by noticing those moments of self-doubt when they arise. It is here that the use of positive affirmations can be very useful. Often we find that our three biggest enemies are "Me,

Myself and I." The limitations that get dumped on us from an early age get internalized, so we then have to deal with internal as well as external "Dream Busters." So who and what are they? In this book, you'll learn why staying mentally healthy is very important and how to build resilience in a stressful world.

CHAPTER 1

WHAT IS MENTAL IMMUNITY?

G lobal pandemic aside, this is the time of year when we start thinking about our physical health. We give up smoking or drinking, commit to daily exercise, January is synonymous with a natural urge to improve our body's strength, immunity, and resilience, even when we're not in the grip of a devastating health crisis.

But when was the last time you thought about your emotional resilience? In the same way that a strong physical immune system can help protect you from illness and encourage a swift recovery when you do become unwell, a strong mental immune system can support you through life's inevitable ups and downs – making you both less susceptible to slumps, and more resilient when things don't go your way.

Mental immunity is our mind's ability to cope with whatever life throws at it. It's about having the capacity to understand, observe and move through painful thoughts or events without either being completely derailed or ignoring them altogether. Good mental immunity is not only about surviving when things get hard, though, but it also requires you to learn and grow from difficult times too.

When we train our minds to expect fearful thoughts or external challenges and tolerate them when they occur, we develop mental immunity. It's about changing one's life goal from avoiding pain to creating meaning while acknowledging that pain will always be a part of the journey.

Life is not easy for anyone. And without healthy emotional resilience, things can start to feel unfathomably tough. Fear, loneliness, change, uncertainty, grief – without a strong foundation, these feelings will threaten to overwhelm you. Life will seem like it's forever knocking you down. And in the same way that a cold or virus can seriously affect the health of someone who is already unwell, even a small setback or upsetting encounter can do the same to someone who lacks mental immunity.

What Is Emotional Resilience?

You can learn a lot about people by seeing how they react to stressful, sad, or even traumatic situations. Do they panic or get angry? Do they shut down? It turns out our ability to cope with adversity is called emotional resilience, and the good news is, if you're intentional, it's a trait you can build and improve over time.

Emotional resilience is an art of living that is entwined with self-belief, self-compassion, and enhanced cognition. It is how we empower ourselves to perceive adversities as 'temporary' and keep evolving through the pain and sufferings.

Emotional resilience is the ability to cope with something healthily and constructively. It's not an outcome but rather a series of attitudinal and behavioral choices for dealing with trauma, tragedy, or other significant life stress.

While people can become more emotionally resilient through experiences later in life, Parmely specifies that building emotional resilience tends to start when we're children. That's right, all those times your parents let you figure something out instead of giving you the answers right away paid off. However, emotional resilience can also be strengthened later in life by facing different struggles and learning from each of them.

How Do Emotions Affect Immunity?

Many studies have shown that chronic exposure to stress, anxiety, and negative moods generally can affect physical health to a large extent.

Scientists are finding more and more proof of the remarkable way our emotions can affect our immune system. When it comes to our health, **there are essentially four things under our control:**

- The decision not to smoke.
- A commitment to exercise.
- The quality of our diet.
- Our level of optimism.

And optimism is at least as beneficial as the others. But, of course, scientists don't yet fully understand the biological mechanisms at work. Still, they know that negative feelings like stress, sadness, and worry cause a spike in the hormone cortisol, suppressing the immune system.

How Your Emotions Affect Your Body

There is a connection between mind and body. Poor emotional health can weaken your body's immune system, making you more likely to get colds and other infections. Our body responds to the way we think, act, and feel. Some symptoms such as headaches, diarrhea, insomnia, palpitations, shortness of breath, loss or weight gain, chest pain, among other symptoms, maybe experienced after an emotional crisis or period of stress like the death of a loved one or being laid off from your job. Also, Psychosomatic illnesses may act upon the health of the body intensely.

The pituitary gland, which connects with the hypothalamus area in the brain, is responsible for the mechanism that triggers diseases since it produces hormones that control all bodily functions.

The hypothalamus perceives the strongest emotions and feelings; these emotions alter the functions of the hypothalamus and its connection to the pituitary gland. Respiratory, skin, circulatory and gastrointestinal diseases caused or aggravated by nervous tension result from this change. Therefore, we can say that psychosomatic illness is emotional problems that cause a psychological component, the manifestation of organic diseases.

How Do You Become Emotional Immune?

As you boost your body's defenses, you can also train your mind to be more resilient. Each of us has an emotional immune system, a set of psychological mechanisms to keep us resilient in the face of adversity, he told me. And like your physical immune system, it's something that can be strengthened.

Understanding the emotional immune system helps to think about how your body responds to germs: A strong immune system doesn't just protect you from pathogens; it's also your body's way of getting you better when you're sick.

It's that second function that applies here. The goal isn't to bat away sadness, fear, or loneliness — that's an impossible task. Instead, your emotional immune system can help you live with those feelings and get yourself to a better place when they come flooding in.

It has never been a more important thing to cultivate. Even those of us who aren't feeling emotionally "sick" by now are pretty run down.

Being emotionally resilient goes beyond merely making it through something hard. It's not just surviving when the dragon comes into our lives but growing from it. When folks are resilient, they're more likely to come out of the other side stronger, wiser, and better.

How to Use Emotional Immunity

Emotional growth might not feel so fun. If you've ever been stuck in bed, burning up with a fever, you know how miserable it is. But that part of the sickness is an essential part of the process. Your body is heating up so you can heal.

The same is true for when you're emotionally run down. To make it through — and grow from — a difficult experience, you have to let the proverbial fever run its course.

- *Take time to grieve.*

Part of resilience is grieving the things you've lost. Say out loud how unfair it is that you lost your job or can't see your loved ones. Admit how much it sucks that you're juggling remote work with caring for a kid. Scream into a pillow if you don't have words.

Whatever you do, you're giving yourself much-needed space to process.

It's so important to take time to understand the breadth and depth of the losses you're experiencing. If you give yourself the chance to process now, at the moment, then you'll be more ready to handle the next painful experience whenever it hits.

- *Be an observer.*

Processing your emotions means letting them get big and overwhelming. It might be tempting to numb yourself against what you're feeling, whether that's with a few glasses of wine or some zoned-out Instagram scrolling, but resist that urge. If you try to skip over the hard parts, you might prolong them.

The premise of mindful acceptance is to identify your thoughts, feelings, and experiences without changing them. For example, acknowledge that you're angry right now, or sad, or afraid; the next time that emotion hits, you'll be able to think back on the last time you made it through.

It's about fortifying your psychological strengths, so when hard things do come your way, you have resources available within you. You don't have to love your emotions, but don't run from them. We're living in a supercharged stressful time on steroids, so whatever you're feeling is very understandable.

Whether you're in the midst of a global pandemic or just having a gloomy day, it's not always possible to fend off pain. But with the right tools, at least you can emerge stronger and more resilient.

Resilience – What Is It And Why?

Do you remember the Weebles and their catchphrase, 'Weebles wobble, but they don't fall down? However much you knock them over, they always bounce back up. For me, that encapsulates resilience - they always finish upright, however many knocks they take, however hard they are hit. What does that mean for humans, though?

Some people like to believe that life will be straightforward. The very idea of life coaching can suggest to people that you can make life what you want it to be, and many coaches will sell their services on that basis. This is not completely true, though, because however well you predict your future, there will always be unanticipated difficulties at various levels of importance. Unexpected grief, not quite hitting your targets, an exam failure; these are all things that can blindside you and knock you down.

Resilience is typically defined as the capacity to recover from difficult life events. Resilience is the ability to withstand adversity and bounce back from difficult life events. Being resilient does not mean that people don't experience stress, emotional upheaval, and suffering. Some people equate resilience with mental toughness, but demonstrating resilience includes working through emotional pain and suffering.

Resilience is the ability to deal with the issue successfully and rise again to carry on. Note that it's not a talent for ignoring the problem. That is a short-term fix that will usually come back to bite you later. Instead, resilience is processing the negative feelings, healing the hurts, putting the pieces back together, and finding a solution that allows you to move on.

Where do the issues come from?

- *Yourself.*

However great you are, there will be times when you make poor choices and then have to suffer the consequences. It might be something simple like that last drink that you didn't need causing you to be hungover at work the next day. It could be more serious, like jumping into a relationship (in work or life) that ultimately doesn't benefit either side. I'm sure you can remember times when you looked back and realized that a problem was of your own making and therefore probably avoidable. For me, these are the hardest to deal with because along with the problem comes the admission that I am not as brilliant as I would like to think! I am plagued with 'what if' scenarios that can easily descend into metaphorical self-flagellation.

- *Others.*

There are also bad events resulting from someone else's actions; these are even less predictable than the results of our actions. This doesn't presume that the people are malicious. Maybe the consequences were completely hidden from them, or possibly they made choices as badly as you sometimes have. However, it might be that your problems stem from the deliberate, possibly criminal, actions of others. Our newspapers are full of such stories.

Why Be Resilient?

Things will go wrong in life. This fact should not be a surprise, even if the actual event is. As you read about the different kinds of issues, you will already have been processing why resilience would help you be better. Being resilient and coping well with the change is the secret to not letting the change derail you for too long. The quicker you can get to a new way of life that works for you, the better. The longer you leave things unresolved, the harder they will be to tackle and the more affected you will be by them. So, assuming you want a bit more success, happiness, or quality of life, stand up and deal with them now. Achieving your goals in life will require you to be resilient and tackle the challenging bits. Some of them can be anticipated and planned around. Others can be avoided by better decision-making on your part, but other obstacles are unavoidable and will need to be overcome.

The alternative is to not deal with them, either not well or not at all, and the consequences become longer lasting and have a bigger negative effect. You can see this in the news where people have become bitter and sad because of past events that affected their lives adversely many years before. But, unfortunately, they never dealt with it, and it is still impacting their lives.

The other possible consequence of not being resilient is that you start to worry. You recognize that problems will occur but become anxious at the thought that you won't be able to deal with them - if you get hit, you will be knocked down and stay there. Many people in this situation will make complex plans to avoid any possible problem, expending huge amounts of mental effort to ensure nothing ever touches them. Unfortunately, this takes a lot of time away from pursuing what should be their main goals in life; instead, they have substituted 'avoiding bad things' as their goal, which will never achieve more.

Resilience can sustain successful performance in the face of adverse conditions, misfortunes, and changes, bounce back, and live life to the full once more. Without it, we condemn ourselves to be in the thrall of the change, controlled by it, rather than taking control of ourselves.

Resilience is important because it gives people the strength needed to process and overcome hardship. Those lacking resilience get easily overwhelmed and may turn to unhealthy coping mechanisms. Conversely, resilient people tap into their strengths and support systems to overcome challenges and work through problems.

Being Resilient – What Skills and Attitudes You Need

It is all very well understanding resilience and acknowledging the need for it, but what is involved in being resilient? We know that we want to be resilient, don't we, but often don't know what that entails. This chapter unpacks some of the ideas around being more resilient. It looks at the skills and attitudes required to cope with the slings and arrows of outrageous fortune, not to mention the deliberate and accidental consequences of people's actions, which have been with us the whole of life.

Several themes appear that are common to many if not all of the writing. These will be described in more detail below but relate to your emotional health, how well you focus on yourself, how well you focus outward and deal with the world, your resiliency skills, and what the resiliency center calls 'a talent for serendipity' (basically your ability to make your own luck)

Emotional health

This is a subject that has been written on at length in recent years. It is one of the basic building blocks for success in any realm because if we are not emotionally healthy, we will struggle to stay in control during the ups and downs of life. This is not to say that we are unemotional or that we don't show our emotions. Instead, it is about being appropriate in our emotionality, not letting things get too extreme. We are allowed to feel sad, to be overjoyed, to weep in grief, to get angry at injustice. How much we let these things take over and rule our lives is what to look for. Being emotionally stable is the aim since this allows us to cope better when things get tough.

Focussing Inward

This is about realistically assessing who you are and what is possible. It is not just trying to put a brave face on things and telling yourself you can get through it. Instead, this stage is about recognizing the weaknesses but also noticing the positives about who you are. What are your personality strengths, particularly those which come into play when times are hard? What is it about you that is useful and good? It might be that you say, 'I am strong' or 'I am trusting' - whatever it is, acknowledge your strengths.

Related to who you are in the step of acknowledging what you can do. Again, be realistic because overly optimistic people aren't the most resilient. How you can cope well in tricky situations is good to know. Besides giving you confidence beforehand, you can proceed during the situation without second-guessing and doubt yourself. To say, 'I can react positively even when I am sad' is good to know. Likewise, knowing you can think clearly through the tears is also useful. What are you capable of?

Finally, within this section, I would include things you have around you that help you deal with events. It might be that you recognize a support network of friends and family that you can go to; it might be that you only identify one close friend. Who is close (however you define that), who can you go to for support? As well as friends, it might be organizations that you have access to. For example, we often forget how lucky we are to call for an ambulance if something goes badly wrong, in the knowledge that a professional will help us. There might be other structures in place to help you too. In the same way that every schoolchild knows exactly what to do when the fire alarm goes off, so we too have ways of dealing with things in emergencies. They might be laid out in company policy, or possibly a way of working that is tried and tested for you; you know it has positive results, so it will kick back into this mode when required.

Focusing Outward

If you are emotionally stable and know yourself well, then the next step is to focus outward and deal with whatever obstacle you have come across. **This is about three things: problem-solving, decision making, and adaptability.**

- *Adaptability.*

Resilience focuses on adaptability, and it is certainly key to dealing with a change in front of you - you could argue that this is indeed the heart of being resilient. Some of this is about simply accepting that things will be different now - the first step in any grief process - and so you will have to be too. It might also involve you doing things differently. Being willing to leave your traditions and old ways is vital to deal with a new situation, even though, on reflection, you recognize that what you did before may still work. The willingness to make changes is vital.

- *Problem-solving.*

This starts with acknowledging that a solution might exist,

followed by a decision that you want to find it. If you merely see the problem and let it overwhelm you, you are not resilient. Instead, searching for the solution and trying things that might make a situation better is the key. You might not solve the whole issue in one go, but making life even a little bit better is a start, as well as an encouragement to carry on trying.

- *Decision-making.*

You noticed in the previous paragraph a decision that had to be made - actually to tackle the problem. The other area is in which direction to go. In problem-solving, you want to develop lots of possible solutions - the more ideas, the better. However, if you simply sit and look at the possibilities and do nothing, you will get nothing. The consequence of indecision is a failure. So deciding for or against a course of action is vital. You don't necessarily need to develop the perfect solution, but you need to decide to act.

Skills

Several skills or attitudes seem to be common to survivors, i.e., resilient people, that seem to help.

- **Reason**

Looking at a bad situation logically and methodically, setting aside emotion, allows you to work through a solution. Panic gets you nowhere. Being realistic and looking simply at facts is what works.

- *Focus.*

It is easy to let ourselves drift off and fantasize about rescue from whatever bad situation we face. Alongside reason sits the ability to focus, being 100% present in the moment. Devoting all your energies to finding a solution makes it more likely that you will find one. It also prevents you from dreaming about being saved, the possibility of which will remove your motivation to work hard for yourself.

- *Humor.*

Being able to find something funny will help. How often have people said, 'If I didn't laugh, I would cry' and is it true? Crying will more likely drag you down towards despair; humor distracts you and lifts your spirits. So allowing yourself to be amused is okay and even beneficial.

- *Integration.*

After the event, it is tempting to box off the tragedy or hardship and never revisit it, sticking it in a mental cupboard. If you have dealt with it successfully, though, it will become as much a part of who you are and what you have become as any other life experience, and probably one that has taught you more than most. Accepting it and integrating the experience and lessons into your life is another factor in being a successful survivor in the future. Pretending it didn't happen, suppressing or ignoring the memories, suggests that you've not dealt with it well.

- *Luck.*

They say people make their own luck, but this is more about simply noticing the 'luck.' Some people notice when 'lucky' things happen to them. In every cloud, they sat there is a silver lining, and if you can find something good out of all that is happening, even after the event, you can accept it more easily.

Being resilient is about who you are before encountering the obstacle and knowing yourself, your strengths, and your support resources. How healthy you are physically and emotionally is important and how you have dealt with your previous life experiences. Resilience is also affected by how you choose to react when you get knocked down; using logic and adapting to deal with the problem well is vital. Being able to laugh about things is useful too. After the event, putting it all in perspective, seeing the bigger picture is vital to your store of 'survival' experiences that will feed into the next occasion.

CHAPTER 2

ALL ABOUT RESILIENCE

How resilient do you think you are? How easily do you bounce back when bad things happen? Do you think you would manage if disability or serious illness were to come your way, or do you think you would buckle under the misery and give up on life? People sometimes say, 'I don't know what I would do if.' But people do manage, somehow life goes on, and for some, their lives are more satisfying and meaningful than previously. So you are probably more resilient than you think you are.

I feel confident of your resilience when I reflect on the children I once worked with. They all had physical disabilities, and many of them faced some amazingly complex issues. Yet 99% of these children showed incredible resilience; they got on with their day-to-day life working hard in school, making friends, enjoying life. Their resilience was taken for granted -- the ones that stood out were those who struggled to cope. It seems that resilience is not a rare trait but something we are all capable of.

Being resilient means being able to cope under stress or pressure or when difficulties come your way. These problems can vary in their enormity: being in a serious accident, facing a natural disaster, not getting a promotion, or even just missing the bus. In life, bad things happen. However, I think knowing you will bounce back means you have already won half the battle. Of course, you may believe you are not the resilient type, so what follows are tips to help you strengthen your resilience and recognize this capability within you.

How do you manage when difficulties come your way? Recall things in your past and what you did to overcome them. Could you have done things differently so you recovered sooner? Note times when you've bounced back in the past. Build on these experiences to help you persevere on your next challenge.

Make sure you know how to recognize and manage your stress. When you feel stress hitting you, two of the easiest ways to help you feel better are exercise and deep breathing. If you are the efficient type, try Yoga as this combines the two.

Have the courage to get support. Being able to turn to others for help is also a sign of resilience. Get support from friends, family, and the community. Today, the community is worldwide thanks to the internet.

When problems come your way, rather than getting over-whelmed with emotion, take on a problem-solving approach. Seek out realistic and attainable solutions that can be quickly implemented.

Recognize how much control you have over how you think and feel and how this impacts your subsequent behavior. Be careful how you define yourself. Don't label yourself a victim. It reduces the amount of control you feel you have. You do not have to be a casualty of your circumstances, and earlier life events do not have to derail you. Studies have shown examples of children growing up in difficult circumstances -- extreme poverty, parents with mental illness or alcoholism - yet they continued to thrive and do well in school.

Learn an optimistic way of thinking. Know that although things may be tough now, at some point, things will be better. Recognize that bad things in life will happen, but start to learn that you will get through them. Be ready for the challenge rather than expect to be defeated. See change as an opportunity rather than something to fight against.

The 7 Components of Resilience

Mental health encompasses far more than the mere absence of disorders. There are several dimensions when it comes to positive mental health, one of which is resilience.

Resilience is the capacity of a system, be it an individual, a forest, a city, or an economy, to deal with change and continue to develop. It is about how humans and nature can use shocks and disturbances like a financial crisis or climate change to spur renewal and innovative thinking.

Resilience is the process of being able to adapt well and bounce back quickly in times of stress. This stress may manifest as family or relationship problems, serious health problems, problems in the workplace, or even financial problems, to name a few.

Developing resilience can help you cope adaptively and bounce back after changes, challenges, setbacks, disappointments, and failures. How do you know if YOU are resilient? **See if you have the following attributes when problems bombard you:**

• *Rebound ability.*

Resilient people bounce back after disasters, shocks,

disappointments, struggles, conflicts, and loss. Refusing to be beaten, they're like kids who fall off a bike and climb on again. Memories of a bad experience? Of course. But the anticipation of great things yet to come overshadows the negative. Hope for something different and better lies in rebound ability.

- *Strength.*

Resilience involves a certain amount of mental, emotional, and physical toughness. This form of toughness leads to durability. It allows a person to resist the permanent devastation of strain in the same way a bullet bouncing off a law enforcement officer's metal vest saves his/her life. Durability results from choosing to expend energy in ways that promote healing, facilitate recovery, and preserve sanity. There is power in exercising strength. This power gives resilient people greater personal control.

- *Centeredness.*

In general resilient individuals are well-grounded psychologically and spiritually. It's hard for people to stay intact if they aren't intact before crisis hits. Imagine trying to locate an inn along a dark country road without an address or phone number. To cope with difficulties, people need to be sure of who they are during stable, more normal times. Such grounding provides a map for finding one's way back to the center after serious challenges, loss, frustration, or pain.

- *Humor.*

Resilience includes a little or a lot of humor. The ability to be in the middle of a situation-or at the end of it and perceive the amusing elements is a gift. Understanding how comical the human condition is, allows folks to see something funny even in a tragedy. While there may not be anything funny about a relative's funeral, there could be some tiny incident, some story, some funny remark, and stands apart from the sadness like a speck of silver glitter on a sheet of black paper.

- *Flexibility.*

One of the best ways to stock the resiliency bank is to learn to adjust to various circumstances rather than resist them. Resistance often brings breakage. People don't have to like their problems, but they may want to embrace them instead of fighting them. With fighting and resisting comes rigidity, and this serves no one. Flexibility implies elasticity, a willingness to flow with whatever happens. Flexible people get sick less and suffer less in the long run.

- *Growth conscious.*

When people are open to possibility, they know that all problems can enhance personal/professional growth. Painful as they may be, the challenges of life shape us one way or another. Why not allow them to mature us, soften us, strengthen us, and remake us into better, more capable human beings? No one ever completes the growing process during a lifetime. Each of us is constantly evolving. To view problems, pain, and loss as opportunities is a sign of moving forward along that continuum.

- *Gratitude.*

Resilient people feel thankful for every event in their lives: the good and joyful and the negative and upsetting. They grasp the fact that all of these together serve as necessary teachers. A grateful heart can be cultivated over time if folks don't have one naturally. It's worth the effort, too, because bitterness cannot coexist with gratitude. Gratitude refreshes the human spirit, gives room for hope, and smoothes away rough edges.

The biggest benefits from developing resilience? Fewer emotional scars. Less anger and fatigue. Enhanced health and deeper joy. New skills. And yes, job preservation perhaps over and over again. However, there's a significant price to pay for leaving resilience out of one's toolbox.

Reasons to Mind Your Emotions

Courage doesn't always roar. Sometimes courage is the little voice at the end of the day that says, 'I'll try again tomorrow.'

Developing emotional resilience and deeper self-awareness has supported me in achieving my goals better, communicating, working with, leading people more effectively, and spring back emotionally after suffering through difficult and stressful times in my life.

Through much searching, reading, listening, practice, and self-reflection, I understand that emotions are never right or wrong, good or bad, or correct or incorrect. Emotions are simply pieces of information telling us how we are currently experiencing our world. However, what we do with the emotions we experience can help or hinder us.

Developing Emotional Resilience

The first step to becoming more emotionally resilient is acknowledging that there is room for improvement and taking the time to learn more about yourself. **The following behaviors and attitudes are some ways in which emotional resilience can be demonstrated and measured:**

- Have realistic and attainable expectations and goals.
- Show good judgment and problem-solving skills.
- Be persistent and determined.
- Be responsible and thoughtful rather than impulsive.
- Be an effective communicator with good people skills.
- Learn from past experience so as not to repeat mistakes.
- Be empathetic towards other people (care how others around you are feeling).
- Have a social conscience (care about the welfare of others).
- Feel good about yourself as a person.
- Feel like you are in control of your life.
- Be optimistic rather than pessimistic.

Some Strategies to develop your Emotional Resilience

There are many strategies we can use to help us harness the positive power of our emotions. **Here are a few for you to consider:**

The Big 4: 7-8 hours of Sleep, Healthy Diet, Regular Exercise, Doing Fun Activities

Relaxation: Learning how to relax takes practice; however, two ways to start is to 1) use progressive Muscle Relaxation or 2) lie still in a warm, safe environment and play quite relaxing music or be in nature - sit quietly, focusing on and experiencing pleasant sensory sensations such as the fragrance flowers or the twittering of birds.

Thought Stopping: As you notice yourself saying something negative in your mind, you can stop your thought mid-stream by saying to yourself, "Stop." Saying this aloud will be more powerful and make you more aware of your habit.

Thought Diary: Keeping a daily diary or journal of your thoughts can be an effective tool for examining your inner process.

Positive Mantras & Affirmations: An affirmation is a positive thought or statement that you repeat to yourself and implant into your unconscious mind. A positive affirmation can act as the source of direction and inspiration for your present and future actions. Once entrenched in your subconscious mind, a positive affirmation guides your thoughts and actions in the desired direction. It can be used to overcome negative and habitual thought patterns to create shifts in your behavior and actions at an unconscious level. Positive affirmations can subtly but pervasively change your self-talk from negative to positive.

Change Self-Limiting Statements to Questions: Self-limiting statements like "I can't handle this!" or "This is impossible!" are particularly damaging because they increase your stress in a given situation. They stop you from searching for solutions. The next time you find yourself thinking something that limits the possibilities of a given situation, turn it into a *q*uestion. Doesn't "How can I handle this?" or "How is this possible?" sound more hopeful, and open up your imagination to new possibilities?

Meditation & Mindfulness: The purpose of meditation is to heal and transform. Because meditation is a skill, you can practice meditation anywhere at any time. In every moment, you can choose to meditate. The energy that crafts and guides the practice of meditation is mindfulness. Mindfulness allows us to look deeply and move beyond the busyness of our minds. It allows us to focus on an object with single-pointed attention. When mindful, we are focused and not distracted.

Five business reasons to Mind Your Emotions

- Healthier, more productive business relationships
- Better staff engagement, alignment, and retention
- Healthy conflict management strategies which address the issues and don't attack the person
- More effective leadership, teamwork, sales, and service outcomes
- Less sick leave, stress claims

Five reasons to Mind Your Emotions

- Self Awareness and Personal Growth
- To experience more positive emotions and less distress in your life
- To increase wanted behaviors and decrease unwanted ones
- To be an effective leader, partner, parent, friend, team player, etc.

- To manage the effect of emotions on personal/team performance, workplace well-being, and happiness.

Mastering Emotions: Taking Your Life To The Next Level

To master emotions and be happy is the ambition of every person. Emotions are the energized feelings. A person cannot avoid emotions since it an impulsive response to circumstances. Emotions include a wide variety of feeling such as fear, guilt, anger, and unworthiness. Anyhow, emotions will impair a person's happiness when the person gets affected by the flood of emotions. Therefore, to maintain a happy outlook, it has become essential to control emotions.

Emotions become most dangerous, when it affects the peoples, interacting with you. In the events of uncontrolled emotion, it is common that it results in outraged behavior and may hurt others' feelings. Thus emotions are a sequential action, which in effect, may badly affect the whole society. The history of humanity shows that many of the black marks happened because of any single emotional outbreak. Therefore, mastery over emotions is essential because it will help you better mold as a good human being.

As told, avoidance of emotions is not practical in daily life; a person can only control emotions. The first step to control the emotions has to begin with the realization of the emotions. You have first to make up your mind to control your emotions. Remember, emotions become dangerous when you react to the impulse. The basic thing to be happy about is to prevent your response. The repeated thought process and regular reminding will restrict your outspoken nature. However, be cautious and seek the advice of the experts while getting started since the suppression of the feelings may cause any other sort of mental disturbances. It is also advisable to a primary investigation about the person's behavior since, in many cases, emotional outbreaks are caused because of mental disorders.

The practice of mental relaxation techniques is an ideal way to control emotions. Relaxation techniques such as meditation, Yoga, biofeedback, and innovative therapies will help relax your mind and keep your mind in your control. Religious faith is also a major factor that can give you consciousness. Involvement in your favorite sports and arts is also a preferred method, which will relax both mind and body. Some recent studies show that diet plays a role in emotional outbreaks, and hence, you have to practice a balanced diet. The step-by-step self-control exercise is focused on remolding the persons for a problem-free and happy life.

Being happy is the intention of everyone. For that, keep in mind an old saying, which means, if you want to be happy, keep others happy. Hence, stop for a moment when you get in touch with anything that raises your emotions. Then, take a deep breath and think about the details of the issue. It is sure that, if you can spare a moment to rethink, you can progress to mastering your emotions and be a very happy person.

Mental Self-Defense Strategies: Reinforcing Your Mental Immune System

What would you do if you felt physically or emotionally threatened in some way? Do you trust your ability to escape a dangerous situation without harm? Would you remain calm and grounded, responding if needed appropriately, or do you fear you'd panic — making a frightening situation worse?

The ability to respond to danger and protect yourself both physically and mentally from violence and fear is a valuable life skill. Especially in these times of uncertainty, protest, and unrest, simply knowing you have the tools to respond in the case of a physical or mental assault can bring peace of mind and boost your self-confidence — even if you never have to use them.

Especially in these times of uncertainty, protest, and unrest, simply knowing you have the tools to respond in the case of a physical or mental assault can bring peace of mind and boost your self-confidence — even if you never have to use them.

Self-defense is not just physical: Mental health can be difficult to talk about objectively, as there is so much emotion and ego involved. One thing to remember is that you are not alone. Many interconnected factors contribute to a mental health breakdown. So defend yourself by taking action!

Mental self-defense is a term used to describe someone protecting themselves from inflicting severe psychological injury - essentially stopping those who influence and manipulate people's minds to serve their self-interest. Mental self-defense encompasses many topics, from a battered woman to corporate marketing and commercials to religious extremism. Essentially anyone trying to use manipulative tactics to influence your decision unconsciously.

Mental Self-Defense & Vulnerabilities

We are all vulnerable to manipulative tactics because we are all human. However, some people are naturally more immune than others. Mental Self Defense aims to help protect individuals and families from becoming victims of deceit, bankruptcy, and death. Most self-proclaimed descendants of god use many manipulative tricks to influence your conscious and unconscious mind. However, if you can stand back and objectively rationalize an argument without becoming emotionally involved, you are one step closer to being left alone.

When a person or group promises to supply a need or want that you desire, he/she will be in a position to manipulate you. **The types of needs may include, but are not limited to the following:**

- A sense of security and belonging or community
- A sense of status within a group
- Being emotionally connected to others or being intimate

Activities To Build Self Esteem

Building your self-esteem is a lifelong process. There are many factors in life that can affect your self-image. It is important to have healthy self-esteem to succeed in all aspects of life. To build self-esteem, **here is advice you can follow:**

Make lists.

One of the most effective ways to build self-esteem is by making lists that contain positive reinforcement about your sense of self. It is helpful to read them over from time to time to feel better about yourself. Having a journal is helpful for this type of exercise.

What to Make Lists of: Just as important as making lists is making significant points that will help boost self-confidence.

- Think of several of your strengths, such as being personable, reliable, brave, or creative.
- List several traits you admire about yourself. For

example, are you a good parent, do you possess spirituality, or make a good effort at your job?

- Think of key achievements in your life, such as graduating from high school or college, landing a successful career, or becoming a wonderful homemaker.
- List several accomplishments completed throughout life, such as learning how to ride a bike, advancing in a degree, or learning a new art or craft.
- Think of at least 10 ways to treat yourself free and do not include food. It could be going for a nature hike or bike ride, playing with your children at the park, or talking with a friend.
- Then think of 5-10 ways to make yourself laugh, help others, and that makes you feel good about yourself.

Reinforce a Constructive Image.

Here is an exercise you can do to build self-esteem. You will need paper, a timer, and a pencil. First, you will set the timer for 10 minutes. Then you need to think about any positive things you can think of yourself, such as a talent or achievement. Everything needs to be positive, though. The thoughts do not need to be organized; they just need to come out on paper as you think of them. Once the 10 minutes are up, you need to read over the list and do this several times a day to reinforce how wonderful a person you are. It is even more effective if read aloud.

Building Optimistic Affirmations.

An affirmation is a statement that you make about yourself to feel better about your self-image. These need to be statements that describe how you would like to feel about yourself over a matter of time. They should not describe how you currently feel about yourself. **Here are some examples of positive affirmations you can say to yourself:**

- I will take care of myself by eating correctly, exercising, doing activities I enjoy, staying in good health, and taking care of myself hygienically.
- I will spend *q*uality time and surround myself with people who treat me well and help me feel good about myself.
- I am a great person who deserves to be here, and some people like and care about me.

If you make your list like the one above and keep it in an accessible place like a wallet or purse, it will be easier to take out and read from time to time. It is best to make copies and keep them in different places that are easy to find. Once you feel confident enough, you may want to share this list with others, although it is perfectly fine not to. As these are read to oneself over and over again, they will become more believable.

Positive Reception Exercise.

Another helpful exercise is the positive reception exercise. On a piece of paper, you will write, "I like (name) because." You will give this paper to friends and family and have them write what they like about you. The point is to not object to anything being written about yourself, just to accept the praise gladly. Again, these are statements you will need to read repeatedly and keep in a place where they can be pulled out and looked at frequently.

You can't learn how to swim from a drowning man. So think about this: are these people who have something to offer, or just people with so much to say and nothing to offer themselves?

You are a power unto yourself, and nobody can truly take that away. Only when we allow other people power over our dreams can we hand over the keys to our future.

Stress and Your Immune System: 10 Ways to Relax and Rejuvenate

Stress seems to have become a constant factor in today's fast-paced society. If left unchecked, it can wreak havoc upon our health. Learning how to manage stress effectively can mean the difference between being robust and full of life or becoming susceptible to illness and disease. Stress can weaken the immune system and accelerate the aging process. The ability to relax and rejuvenate promotes wellness, vitality, and longevity.

A healthy immune system regulates our body's healing process and protects it against infections and diseases. When stress compromises our immune function, it can result in colds, flu, fatigue, cardiovascular disorders, and premature aging. This is because stress increases heart rate, blood pressure, glucose levels, adrenaline, cortisol, free radicals, and oxidative damage. This initiates the "fight or flight" response, places undue strain upon the heart, and increases anxiety and depression.

Protecting the immune system is a vital part of living longer, feeling younger, and being healthy. **Here are ten natural healthy** ways to reduce stress, boost your immune system and slow down the hands of time:

- **Walking and Physical Activity (dancing, gardening, cycling, swimming, etc.).** Regular exercise and physical activity strengthen your immune system, cardiovascular system, heart, muscles, and bones. It also stimulates the release of endorphins, improves mental functioning, concentration/attention, and cognitive performance, and lowers cholesterol, blood pressure, cortisol, and other stress hormones. Three 10-minute workout sessions during the day are just as effective as one 30-minute workout and a lot easier to fit into a busy schedule.
- **Yoga and Stretching.** The slow movements and controlled postures of yoga improve muscle strength, flexibility, range of motion, balance, breathing, blood circulation and promotes mental focus, clarity, and calmness. Stretching also reduces mental and physical stress, tension, and anxiety, promotes good sleep, lowers blood pressure, and slows down your heart rate.
- **Hand Hygiene.** The most effective measure in preventing the spread of microorganisms that cause infections is good hand hygiene. Washing your hands with soap and water as soon as you come home and always before you eat greatly reduces your exposure to bacterial and viral infections. If you cannot wash with soap and water when you are away from home, carry some alcohol-based hand wipes with you to control microbial exposure and transmission.
- **Laughter and Humor.** There is truth to the saying that laughter is the best medicine. Laughing reduces stress

hormones like adrenaline (epinephrine) and cortisol. It also benefits your immune system by increasing the number and activity of Natural Killer T-cells. These cells act as the first line of defense against viral attacks and damaged cells. So find the humor in things and engage in activities that make you laugh to increase your immune function and disease resistance.

- **High Nutrient Diet.** Eat foods rich in antioxidants (like vitamins A, C, E, and lycopene), omega-3 fatty acids, and folate. Antioxidants fight and neutralize free radicals, which damage cells and cause heart disease, cancer, and premature aging. Omega-3 fatty acids (a polyunsaturated fat) have anti-inflammatory, cardiovascular-enhancing, and immune-regulating properties. It helps prevent and control high cholesterol, hypertension, heart disease, stroke, cancer, diabetes, depression, inflammatory and auto-immune disorders. Folate prevents age-related cognitive decline, damage to blood vessels and brain cells by lowering homocysteine levels. It also ensures DNA integrity (important as we age and when pregnant) and promotes healthy red blood cells. **Excellent food sources for these nutrients are as follows:**

Antioxidants - pumpkin, sweet potatoes, carrots, kale, grapefruit (red and pink), blueberries, strawberries, watermelon, cantaloupe, oranges, peppers (red and green), tomatoes, broccoli, sunflower seeds, almonds, and olive oil.
Omega-3 Fatty Acids - ground flax seeds, walnuts, salmon, soybeans, and pumpkin seeds.
Folate - dark green leafy vegetables (turnip greens, mustard

greens, spinach, romaine lettuce, collard greens, etc.), beans, legumes, asparagus, Brussels sprouts, beets, and okra.

- **Music.** Listening to your favorite music is a great method of reducing stress and relieving anxiety. Your individual preference in music determines which types of soothing sounds will best reduce your tension, blood pressure and promote feelings of tranquility. Pay attention to how you feel when you hear a particular song or genre of music, and keep listening to the ones that produce a relaxing effect.
- **Sleep.** Getting enough sound sleep profoundly impacts your stress levels, immune function, and disease resistance. A chronic lack of sleep can leave you feeling sluggish, irritable, forgetful, accident-prone, and have difficulty concentrating or coping with life's daily aggravations. Long-term sleep loss can also result in heart disease, stroke, hypertension, depression, and anxiety. Sleep time is when your body and immune system do most of their repairs and rejuvenation. Strive to get 7-8 hours of sleep each night.
- **Positive Thinking.** Optimism can counteract the negative impact stress, tension, and anxiety have on your immune system and well-being. Often it is how you perceive things that determine if you get overwhelmed, both mentally and physically. Having a positive attitude, finding the good in what life throws your way, and looking at the bright side of things enhance your ability to manage stress effectively.
- **Tea.** Regularly drinking tea throughout the day can help strengthen your immune system and your body's ability to fight off germs and infections. Both green and

black teas contain a beneficial amino acid called L-theanine, which can increase the infection-fighting capacity of gamma delta T cells. L-theanine also promotes a sense of relaxation, calmness, and well-being by influencing the release and concentration of neurotransmitters (like dopamine, serotonin, and GABA) in the brain.

- **Hydrotherapy.** Relaxing in a hot bath relieves sore muscles and joints, reduces stress and tension, and promotes a good night's sleep. Add some soothing music, soft lighting, and naturally scented bath salts or bubble bath/bath foam to create an inexpensive and convenient spa experience in the privacy of your home.

CHAPTER 3

WHY STAYING MENTALLY HEALTHY IS VERY IMPORTANT

When you think of adult health, you may think about various ways to stay healthy - from hand washing and vaccines to cancer prevention. Good for you for making healthy choices daily, which are the stepping stones toward promoting adult health.

It is equally important to pay attention to your signs and symptoms. Know which adult health warning signs merit medical attention, from unexplained weight loss or changes in bowel habits to shortness of breath and sudden headaches.

And, of course, regular physical exams and adult health screening tests are an important part of preventive adult health care. Know which screening tests you need and how often to have them done. Early detection is often the key to successful treatment.

The main health screening guidelines are:

- Blood pressure
- Breast cancer/cervical cancer/prostate cancer/colon and rectal cancer

- Cholesterol
- Dental health
- Diabetes
- Eye health

How can you tell whether a mental health issue is normal or not? It can be tricky. The line between normal and abnormal mental health is often blurred. Still, it is helpful to consider your feelings, thoughts, and behavior related to cultural norms and other benchmarks.

Often, anger management is a key aspect of mental health; expressed appropriately, anger can be healthy. Anger itself is not the problem - it is how you handle it. Consider whether you may benefit from new ways to manage anger.

Mental health also includes issues such as self-esteem, friend-ships, and resilience. If you struggle with self-esteem, denial, or other mental health issues, remember that help is available. To find a mental health provider, ask your family doctor for a referral.

Yes, lack of sleep can affect your immune system. Studies show that people who do not get a good night's sleep or who do not get enough sleep are more likely to get sick after being exposed to a virus, such as the common cold. Lack of sleep can also affect how fast you recover if you do get sick.

During sleep, your immune system releases proteins called cytokines. These substances increase in the presence of an infection, inflammation, and stress. Increased cytokines are necessary for fighting infection and regulating deeper sleep. In addition, other infection-fighting cells are reduced during periods of sleep deprivation. So, your body needs sleep to fight infectious diseases.

How much sleep do you need to bolster your immune system? The optimal amount of sleep for most adults is seven to eight hours a night. However, school-aged children and adolescents need nine or more hours of sleep a night.

But be careful; more sleep is not always better.

For adults, sleeping more than nine to 10 hours a night has been associated with weight gain, heart problems, stroke, sleep disorders, depression, and other health concerns.

Strategies on How To Build Resilience In a Stressful World

Being resilient is not about glossing over hard times and pretending they didn't happen; it's coping with them in a way that allows you to bounce back.

Adopting a positive attitude and developing the right skills in the midst of difficulties is important because they help you live a happy life. You'll be able to achieve your personal goals and have a better relationship with others and yourself.

Do you think you need help building resilience? Are you looking to become calmer? Are you struggling with moving on from a heartbreaking, traumatic, or disappointing experience?

Here are some simple yet valuable strategies for becoming resilient in a stressful world:

- *Focus on what you can control.*

You need to understand one thing: You are not in control of every single thing that happens in your life.

More often than not, we think about what we could have or have not done to prevent a negative event. However, there is no use stressing about something you cannot take back.

Remember this: The only thing you can control is yourself. So put all your anxieties aside.

Ask yourself, "What is the next best thing I can do at this moment to make myself better?" Then do it.

- *Practice an attitude of gratitude.*

Can you identify at least 5 things that are going well in your life at this moment?

Developing an attitude of gratitude changes your perspective, how you look at certain situations. Instead of excessively worrying about what's missing, focus on your blessings. Whether you have food on the table, clean air, a loving spouse or friend, or a career, anything that's good is something worth being thankful for.

If you want to become more appreciative of what you have, meditate on these things. Write them down in a journal. Talk about them! The more you do it, the more it becomes you.

- *Exercise regularly.*

Yes, doing exercise, a daily habit, helps you become more resilient.

Imagine yourself sweating, your heart racing, and your respiratory rate going up when you exercise. They simulate real-life hardships. The more you exercise, the stronger you become physically, emotionally, and mentally.

If you are emotionally sensitive, engaging in regular physical activity builds your resilience. Put in mind that you are way stronger than you imagine.

- *Don't forget to love yourself first.*

When was the last time you took good care of yourself? Do you accept yourself for your strengths and flaws, or are you too self-critical?

You are worthy; always keep that in mind. Self-love is deeply appreciating you for who you are and not imposing unrealistic expectations.

Self-love matters more than you think it does. When you love yourself, you are more likely to be happy and authentic. No one can use your weakness against you.

These are just some of the best ways for you to develop resilience. However, the strategies here will already put you off to a good start. Resilience takes time and a lot of patience, but its benefits for your life are truly worthwhile.

Building Mental Resilience – Seven Secrets to Difficult Times

As difficult economic times drag on, it can get harder and harder to keep a positive attitude. However, keep in mind that the same techniques and life skills can work no matter the circumstances. We, humans, are built to solve problems, and we are meant to be happy!

If a woman loses her job, forecloses on a home, fails a test, or breaks up with a loved one, it can be difficult and depressing. Would you know what to do? When life hands you a bunch of lemons, do you fall apart and spend months trying to recover, or are you resilient? Do you weather the ups and downs to come back stronger, or do you hide under a rock until the storm blows over? During these trying times, it's especially important to be resilient and prepared for anything.

Resilient people are "mentally tough." Think of them like the Energizer Bunny; they keep going and going no matter what. But how can you develop this kind of strength and perseverance? What is their secret?

Resilience is a trait many people possess. Those who are resilient can overcome difficult situations and remain cool, calm, and collected. They are ready to seek solutions and get back on track. They do not let disappointments deter them from what they want. Instead, they stay focused and plan to be successful. We can all learn to be more resilient and mentally tough. It's all about being in the ideal psychological, physical, and emotional state to perform at peak levels. Performance is about how we go about our lives, how we behave, feel, think, do our jobs.

Regardless of where we perform these functions and responsibilities, it is important to know how well we are doing and improve or change. Ask yourself what state you are in. How are you doing with all of these things? Are you happy? Are you pleased with life as it is now?

If you want more out of your life, whether it's to do better on the job, be promoted to the next level, or dedicate more time to your family and friends, then it's time to consider tweaking things to start performing at peak levels.

Here are seven tools to help you become more mentally tough and resilient:

- **Start breathing.** This activity prepares your body for better performance. Are you holding your breath right now? If you are stressed or anxious, you might be not only holding your breathing in, but you could be having headaches, backaches, or tightening shoulders. So here's a prescription for you: Take three deep breaths and let them out slowly. Count one, two, three. This creates good circulation and steady breathing for the rest of your day.

- **Get more physical activity.** Call it exercise or whatever you want. Anything that will get your heart pumping creates important changes in your body. Exercise gives every woman a sense of control, and as we all know, control is important to us as human beings! Physical activities such as running, walking, doing yoga or Pilates, going biking, hiking, swimming, or playing sports are all great ways to keep your mind and body healthy.

- **Give your body the fuel it needs.** Food fuels your human engine. You would not leave the house without putting gas in your car when you are ready to take a long drive, and yet you might not think twice about leaving for work without eating breakfast. Where is the sense in that? Instead, fill up your tank with energy-boosting whole grains, fruits, yogurt and watch your performance increase.

- **Get laughing.** When the going gets tough, the tough start laughing! Go out and find your sense of humor. Whether it's a comedy club, a funny movie, or getting together with a particularly comedic friend, it's time to locate your funny bone and increase those feel-good endorphins. This will help not only with your emotional state but also your physical being. Think about it. When you laugh, you breathe. So try it and do a big belly laugh and see what happens. Have you noticed after a funny movie how much better you feel?

- **Visualize your future.** Practice what you want to be and see clearly what you want for your future. It may seem silly, but practicing in your mind, whether it's a skill you are trying to attain or the dream house you want to move into, can open up new possibilities. Athletes do it all the time. They will visualize the ball going into the hole or the basketball going into the net. Think, and it will be: "This success is mine."

- **Use your brain.** The bottom line is that mentally tough people, resilient people, use their brains. It must be exercised. So, go out there and do brain games. Try out right-brain-left-brain exercises such as puzzles, cards, and memory games; brush your hair (or your teeth) with the opposite hand; find a new way to get home after work; even skipping and jumping rope is right-left brain exercises. We use around 11 percent of our brainpower, which means 89 percent of our brains are waiting to get used. Think of all that potential!

- **Stay cool.** Mentally tough people know how to stay calm and avoid letting their emotions run over them. Here are some tips for that: Try doing some biofeedback; spend the afternoon daydreaming; listen to music; get a fuzzy pet. Last but not least, get rid of those negative thoughts! For example, stop saying "I can't" and replace it with "I can or I will."

Most importantly, resilient, mentally tough women choose to be happy! Happiness is a state of mind, not a place, an object, person, or thing. Think of the Laws of Attraction. You attract what you think. Mentally tough people practice being happy and know it is up to them to make it happen. They also know that practicing makes them good at it. The good news is all of this costs absolutely nothing. You do not have to go and buy a manual or a single piece of expensive equipment.

Times are tough... but the tough get going, and we can learn a lot from them. Be happy and be mentally resilient, and you will be able to handle anything that comes your way!

CHAPTER 4

HOW TO DEVELOP MENTAL RESILIENCE

We all possess some degree of mental strength. But there is always room for improvement. Developing mental strength is about improving your ability to regulate your emotions, manage your thoughts, and behave positively, despite your circumstances.

Just as some are predisposed to develop physical strength more easily than others, mental strength seems to come more naturally to some people.

There are several factors at play to determine the ease with which you develop mental strength:

- *Genetics.*

Genes play a role in whether or not you may be more prone to mental health issues, such as mood disorders.

- *Personality.*

Some people have personality traits that help them think more realistically and behave more positively by nature.

- *Experiences.*

Your life experiences influence how you think about yourself, other people, and the world in general.

Despite these factors that are mostly beyond your control, you can increase your mental strength by devoting time and energy to self-improvement.

To understand mental strength, you have to become aware of how intertwined your thoughts, behaviors, and feelings are, often working together to create a dangerous downward spiral.

Therefore, developing mental strength requires a three-pronged approach. First, we have to manage our thoughts, behaviors, and emotions.

Here are some more specific tips on how to strengthen and manage your thoughts, behaviors, and emotions:

- To strengthen your thoughts, you must identify irrational thoughts and replace them with more realistic ones.
- To strengthen your behaviors, you must strive to behave positively, despite circumstances around you.
- To strengthen your emotions, you must strive to control your feelings and emotions, not to control you.

Psychologists believe that we should always think positively. But, unfortunately, optimism alone isn't enough to help you reach your full potential. What you have to do in addition is to choose behavior based on balanced emotions and rational thinking.

Balancing Emotions and Rational Thinking

We can make our best decisions in life when we balance our emotions with rational thinking. So stop and think for a minute about how you behave when you're really angry. You've likely said and done some things that you regretted later.

However, making choices based on rational thinking alone also doesn't make good decisions. We are human beings and not robots, after all. Our hearts and heads need to work together to control our bodies.

We all have some difficulty controlling our thoughts, emotions, and behavior consistently. However, the more often we control them, the more mentally resilient we will become. And this is a recipe for success.

Six Tips To Build Mental Resilience, Prevent Brain-Damaging Stress, And Improve Brain Health

These days, we all live under considerable stress -- economic challenges, job demands, family tensions, always on technology and the 24-hour news cycle all contribute to ceaseless worry.

While many have learned to simply "live with it," this ongoing stress can, unless properly managed, have a serious negative impact on our ability to think clearly and make good decisions, in the short-term, and even harm our brains in the long-term.

Too much stress can almost make us "forget" how to make changes to reduce that stress, limiting the mental flexibility needed to find alternative solutions and triggering the sensation of "burnout" -- which makes us feel unmotivated and mentally exhausted. This is why, next time you forget someone's name at a party, try not to obsess about remembering it. Instead, make fun of your DNA (we are all human, aren't we). The name in question is then more likely to appear in your mind when you expect it less.

What Can You Do?

Rather than simply living with stress, learning how to effectively master our stress levels and build emotional resilience as part of our brain fitness efforts can not only help you feel and perform better daily but also protect your brain from the long-term damaging effects of stress. **Here's how to do it:**

1. **Get some exercise:** Studies show that aerobic exercise helps build new neurons and connections in the brain to counteract the effects of stress. A study found that people who exercised very little showed greater stress related atrophy of the hippocampus (the part of the brain that stores memories) compared to those who exercised more. Regular exercise also promotes good sleep, reduces depression and boosts self-confidence through the production of endorphins, the "feel-good" hormones.

2. **Relax:** Easier than it sounds, right? But relaxation -- through meditation, tai chi, yoga, a walk on the beach, or whatever helps to quiet your mind and make you feel more at ease -- can decrease blood pressure, respiration rate, metabolism, and muscle tension. Meditation, in particular, is tremendously beneficial for managing stress and building mental resilience.

Studies also show that getting out into nature can have a positive, restorative effect on reducing stress and improving cognitive function. So move your yoga mat out into the yard, or turn off that treadmill and take a walk in the park. Your brain will thank you for it.

3. **Socialize:** When your plate is running over and stress takes over, it's easy to let personal connections and social opportunities fall off the plate first. But ample evidence shows that maintaining stimulating social relationships are critical for both mental and physical health. Create a healthy environment, inviting friends, family and even pets to combat stress and exercise all your brains.

4. **Take control:** Studies show a direct correlation between feelings of psychological empowerment and stress resiliency. Empowering yourself with a feeling of control over your situation can help reduce chronic stress and give you the confidence to take control over your brain health. Some video games and apps based on heart rate variability can be a great way to be proactive and take control of our stress levels.

5. **Have a laugh:** We all know from personal experience that a good laugh can make us feel better, and this is increasingly backed by studies showing that laughter can reduce stress and lower the accompanying cortisol and adrenaline levels that result. Having fun with friends is one way to practice to two good brain health habits at once. Even just thinking about something funny can have a positive effect on reducing stress and the damage it causes to your brain.

6. **Think positive:** How you think about what stresses you can actually make a difference. In a study, students

were coached into believing that the stress they feel
before a test could actually improve performance on
graduate school entrance exams. Compared with
students who were not coached, those students earned
higher scores on both the practice test and the actual
exam. Simply changing the way you look at certain
situations, taking stock of the positive things in your
life and learning to live with gratitude can improve
your ability to manage stress and build brain resilience.
Trying a variety of challenging brain teasers is another
great way to develop mental resilience.

Living with high levels of sustained stress can have a profound
negative impact on your psychological and brain health. While
often there is little we can do to change the stressful situation
itself; there are many things we can do to alter or manage our
reactions to it. Managing stress and mastering our emotions
through simple lifestyle changes and the use of basic techniques
that anyone can do can help reduce stressrelated damage to the
brain, improve emotional resilience and thwart cognitive decline
as we age.

Six Steps To Mental Resilience

Among the vital organs inside your body, your brain is the most
overused. That is because you are doing a lot of thinking when
you perform your tasks or even when you are just taking a good
night's sleep. Your brain does not stop working, and it shouldn't,
or else you will be dead. So expect heavy thoughts and mental
fatigue to come your way, especially if you are a physically and
mentally active person.

When you are making up your plans for healthy living, you

should consider how you can take care of your mental health by focusing on the psychological aspect of wellness.

Here are six steps you can achieve psychological well-being:

1. **Talk to someone.** Sometimes, we strain our thoughts by thinking of all our problems and keeping them within ourselves. You need to let go and speak up your thoughts to someone whom you trust the most. It can be your mom and dad, your friend, or even your pets. Empty your worries through words by telling them what you feel.

2. **Underline your priority goal.** Sometimes it is not the problems that make us anxious or perplexed, but our plans and goals in life. We face a lot of opportunities that we do not know where and when to start. If your goal for today is to lose weight, focus on it first and set aside other plans, such as buying a new car, preparing dinner for friends, or traveling abroad. Implement one plan at a time so that you can accomplish everything without hassles.

3. **Do something pleasurable.** The workplace is a den of different kinds of stressors that make you feel exhausted when you return home. However, you do not have to think too much about workplace stress, especially during weekends or non-working days when you are given some break time. Instead, take your free time as a chance for you to unwind your thoughts by doing your favorite hobby, such as playing a sport, going to the beach, preparing a barbecue party at your yard, watching your favorite movies, or taking care of your pets. All of these pleasurable activities can deviate

your thoughts for a while from all those mind-numbing problems at the workplace.

4. **Exercise your mind.** There are some exercises that are purely intended to relax your thoughts. One of these is yoga. It allows the positive flow of energy in your mind and body that helps relaxes tired muscles and composes your thoughts.

5. **Spend some quality time sleep.** Sleeping is one of the best ways to calm down a bushed mind. It will help regenerate your brain cells' energy, and it also loosens up the heavy load in your mind.

6. **Stay positive.** One of the best ways for healthy living is always to stay positive. No matter how many problems and pressures you face in life, you need to be optimistic. By doing so, you will get rid of apprehensions and worries that hamper you from thinking clearly.

CHAPTER 5

WHAT MAKES YOU HAPPY?

Characteristics of Resilient People

W hat makes you happy? It is easy to stay happy when times are good. However, it is more challenging when life has thrown you a curve.

In difficult times it is important to be resilient. Resilience is that quality that enables people to face adversity and adapt to it without lasting difficulties. A resilient person can "roll with the punches."

Some people are born with more resilience than others. However, we all can become more resilient. Knowing the characteristics of resilient people can help you to become more resilient yourself.

Here are the ten characteristics of resilient people:

1. They are strong people who realize the importance of having a good social support system and can surround themselves with supportive friends and family.

2. They look at the bright side of a situation. They believe in their strength and their ability to address and overcome any problem. During a crisis, they are good to have around because of their optimism.

3. They have a spiritual practice. They have faith in themselves and the universe to overcome anything. (This doesn't mean you can't be resilient if you don't have a spiritual practice. It just means a connection has been found.)

4. They are childlike in their interest in what is going on. They are curious about situations. They experiment, wonder about things, and laugh. They are not caught up in what was (the history). Instead, they focus on the new possibilities.

5. They are connected to what is most important to them in life (their values) and see meaning and purpose in what they do. Instead of getting emotional about a situation, they align their thoughts and actions with their values.

6. They focus on the important things and don't fight things they can not control. Resilient people save their energy to fight the necessary battles. They know what they control and what is out of their reach.

7. They take responsibility for their physical well-being. That allows them to be physically and emotionally resilient. They eat healthy food, exercise, and get enough rest. This buffers them from life's stresses.

8. When a problem arises, they seek solutions. They can live with uncertainty and ambiguity until they find the solution. This gives them room to grow.

9. They always see something negative as an opportunity to do something better or get something

better. They consider adversity a challenge, not a threat.

10. They don't take themselves too seriously. They have a sense of humor about life's challenges.

The Benefits of Mental Strength

It's easy to feel emotionally strong when life is going well. However, we all go through periods of time when our life is going anything but well. There are sickness, death, and injustices that we all face every day regardless of the kind of steps we take to avoid them.

When you are mentally strong, you are much more able to deal with life's challenges. And this will help you to become a better person.

The benefits of increasing mental strength are as follows:

1. **You will experience increased resilience to stress.** Mental strength is helpful in everyday life, not just in the midst of a crisis. As a result, you become better equipped to handle problems more efficiently and effectively, and it can reduce your overall stress levels.

2. **You will experience improved life satisfaction.** As your mental strength increases, your confidence will also increase. You behave according to your values, which will give you peace of mind, and you'll recognize what's important in your life.

3. **You will experience enhanced performance.** Whether your goals are to be a better writer or increase your productivity, increasing your mental strength will help you reach your full potential.

To improve your mental strength, you have to improve every day by developing new ways of dealing with difficulties and using some measures to avoid emotional outbursts as much as possible.

Here are a few ways to try and improve every day:

- Do everything to the best of your ability.
- Don't rush.
- Don't expect improvement fast-instead expect things to be slow yet consistent.
- Try to learn and hone your skills continuously.
- Do things that make you happy and content.
- Don't hang around negative people.
- Take pride in who you are.

By taking these steps, you will be taking additional steps to improve, and when you do, you will gain the self-confidence that you need to plow forward, regardless of what you are trying to achieve.

However, please remember to be patient in this process. It can take a long time to develop increased mental resilience. But, the more patient you are with yourself, the better you will feel, and the more you will achieve. So, slow and consistent will win the race for you.

By taking steps to become increasingly mentally resilient as a writer every day, you will become more successful and excellent over time.

Becoming Mentally Tough To Better Manage Stress

When you are faced with an unexpected challenge or change, how do you normally respond to it? Do you see it as a challenge or an opportunity to stretch your capacity to be more and do more? Your answer to this question can indicate your mental toughness.

Key Factors for Mental Toughness

These factors comprise their 4C Model for overall mental toughness. **They are:**

- **Challenge:** seeing challenge as an opportunity
- **Confidence:** having high levels of self-belief
- **Commitment:** being able to stick to tasks
- **Control:** believing that you control your destiny

Think about a recent incident in which you faced relentless demands, change, or unexpected challenges, on a scale of 1 to 3, with one being bad, two being just o.k., and three being pretty good; how would you score your response to the stress that you felt in the situation? One could argue that a central component of mental toughness is how effective one deals with potentially stressful situations.

A Reason Why Some People Respond Differently to Stress

I'm sure that you have recognized how the people in your sphere of influence manage stress. For example, one person may use stress to "motivate them to thrive in the face of a challenge, while another sees the stressor as a threat," and it seems to take the wind out of their sail.

A reason for this could be based on the trait anxiety theory, "which is the personality factor that predisposes an individual to view certain situations as more or less anxiety-provoking. Individuals with high trait anxiety perceive events as being more threatening than individuals with lower trait anxiety.

A resilient attitude is closely connected to the degree of mental toughness that we exhibit. The stick-to-itiveness factor demonstrates the amount of effort and perseverance we spend on completing tasks and achieving goals. A resilient attitude reflects our internal thinking process, so mental training is not just important for athletes; it's important for you and me.

A Mental Strength Regimen

You can increase your mental toughness by developing resiliency. **Below are the following skills we need to develop to cultivate resiliency and be mentally tough:**

- **Emotional regulation:** Resilient people manage their internal world, which helps them control their emotions, attention, and behavior.
- **Impulse Control:** Resilient people manage the behavioral expression of their emotional impulses, including the ability to delay gratification. Impulse control is correlated with emotional regulation.
- **Causal analysis:** Resilient people can get outside of their habitual thinking styles to identify more possible causes and thus more potential solutions.
- **Self-efficacy:** Resilient people believe in themselves and build others' confidence in them, placing them in line for more success and more opportunity.

- **Realistic optimism:** Resilient people can stay positive about the future without Pollyanna-style optimism.
- **Empathy:** Resilient people can read others' non-verbal cues to help build deeper relationships with them and tend to be more in tune with their emotional state.
- **Reaching out:** Resilient people take on new challenges and opportunities, enhancing the positive aspects of life.

As humans, none of us are going to hit home runs each time we feel stressed. That is an unrealistic expectation from an imperfect vessel. However, we can take a proactive approach to develop our mental toughness so that we aren't so easily miffed every time we encounter a stressor in life.

The way that we approach a circumstance significantly affects how the experience is handled. By developing and nurturing the "mental strength regimen" skills, we can better manage our thoughts, emotions, and behaviors, increase our capacity to manage stress better and improve our well-being and positive behavior toward others.

Five Key Principles of Mental Toughness and Resilience

Throughout our lives, we face change and challenges. Nothing stays the same; the good times don't last, but neither do the bad times. People and places come and go; the world changes, and so does our place within it. To survive the changes, we need to be adaptable and refocus on our objectives. We may have to modify who we are and how we are to face the new realities. We must strive to find opportunity in adversity. Of course, all of this is easier said than done. **Here are the five key principles of mental toughness and resilience:**

- *Rational Thinking.*

We are what we think. When we change our thoughts, we change how we feel and act. Rational thinking and rational beliefs are the foundations of mental toughness and resilience; they assist us in our aims, objectives, and survival. Rational beliefs are flexible and non-extreme; they are based on reality and the available evidence. The emphasis is on seeing things as they are and keeping any negative attributes in perspective and proportion not to overreact emotionally or avoid challenges. If our thinking and beliefs are dogmatic, rigid, or extreme, we remain trapped in the past and are doomed to repeat the same mistakes. The key is to ask ourselves, "how is thinking or behaving this way helping me to feel good or achieve my goals?"

Rational thinking is resilient thinking and helps us build our tolerance for frustration and discomfort without making "mountains out of molehills" or seeing a situation as being worse than it is. The fact is that things could always be worse. Our rational thoughts and beliefs are essential to overcoming unhelpful emotions and behavior such as anxiety, depression, and avoidance. By changing our thinking, we change who we are, how we feel, and what we do.

- *Responsibility.*

Mental toughness means that we take ultimate responsibility for our thoughts, emotions, and behavior, together with responsibility for our decisions and the likely consequences of our actions. Events and conditions will, of course, have an impact and an effect on us, but we are responsible for the things that come within our domain of influence. Events can only upset us if we allow them to. Nothing and no one can bother or disturb us unless we permit them to do so. We choose what we think, how we feel, and what we do.

To be resilient, we need to take responsibility; otherwise, we will tend to view ourselves as pawns and victims. We may blame everyone and everything for our conditions rather than take active steps to change whatever we are capable of. At times we may all seek to blame the government or this or that corporation for the way our lives are, but the ultimate responsibility is still ours. We are ultimately in control.

- *Adaptability.*

For mental toughness and mental health in general, we need to be adaptable. We may seem mentally healthy when we are suited to the conditions around us, such as our jobs, relationships, and home. However, if these conditions change and we cannot adapt, we are at risk of poor mental health. Change is uncomfortable, but we need to accept some discomfort and pain to learn, adapt and survive. If we remain static and fixed in our outlook, the world moves on and leaves us behind.

Resilient people do not see themselves as victims of change. They do not complain "why me" and demand that bad things must not happen to them. Instead, resilient people see bad events as a normal (although unwelcome) part of life; they adjust to the new reality. Evolution favors those who can adapt to new environments and realities; we must be relentless in our adaptability, ingenuity, and creativity to survive. This is true of individuals and organizations.

- *Commitment.*

Mental toughness and commitment have a clear idea of what we want out of life - our goals, objectives, and purpose. If we don't know where we are going, then any road will take us there. It is healthy if our commitments extend to different areas of our lives, such as our relationships, careers, health, and home, rather than focusing on just one or two areas. It is also helpful to be committed to things outside of ourselves, such as charity work, local groups, or political concerns. A key aspect of commitment is that it provides us with meaning in our lives. If we ask ourselves, "What is the meaning of life?" then our commitments and goals should provide the answer.

Having goals and being resilient means that we will keep going and solve problems in the face of setbacks and difficulties. When life knocks us down, we will pick ourselves up again. We will tolerate short-term frustration and discomfort for our long-term gain. Resilience and persistence are key; most people simply give up.

- *Confidence.*

Confidence is our belief in our ability to get things done. Our confidence will vary according to different circumstances and events. For mental toughness and resilience, we need to increase the areas where we feel confident consistently. We may prefer to stay within our comfort zones, but the world changes, and eventually, all comfort zones will become uncomfortable. Our comfort zones become comfort traps.

To be more confident, we need to be accurate in our appraisal of threats. If we perceive that challenges are unrealistically dangerous or threatening, then we will not take action. If we avoid failure, we also avoid success, so we need to take calculated risks and step outside our comfort zones. To be resilient, we need to be less concerned about how others view us and what we believe they are thinking or saying about us. We need to challenge our self-imposed limits and our restricted views of reality. We don't see things as they are; we only see things as we are.

CHAPTER 6

EMOTIONAL RESILIENCY -
THE COURAGE TO OVERCOME
FEAR

For some people, it takes a lot of courage to get up in the morning. It takes courage to try and just survive through another day. I am sure you can think of many people and circumstances in your mind's eye right now that fit that image...from a neighbor down the street to someone on the other side of the world. It's almost impossible to fathom where that person can find such enormous amounts of courage.

Some mornings when we awake, we can see right away that it will be an amazingly clear and spectacular day. The sun hasn't risen yet, but we know it's going to. We can see the light and the lack of clouds in the sky. We can hear a few birds, apparently happy that their nesting isn't going to be interrupted by weather conditions. Yet, we don't feel so good....we don't feel like jumping out of bed and chirping away while we are doing our nesting chores.

There are days that we arise with joy. It is just there inside us, and we look forward to meeting the day even if we see only clouds or rain. There is a sense of well-being, and excitement is in the air. We can see the beauty of life and the potential of the day.

We all have these days. You may be thinking right now about how you felt the same this morning or yesterday morning, or last week. You may be dreading certain things and end up avoiding doing them. Fear and procrastination can certainly cause one to feel even more stress, even though there is temporary relief in one's comfort zone. No matter your economic status or how physically attractive you are, life does not let you escape the ups and downs. So how do you stay motivated when you don't feel so good and hold on to that healthy perspective when life is beautiful? How do you set this example day after day for your children?

We would like to suggest two important ways to approach those difficult days when searching for courage.

The first tip for the doldrums or when you or your children are distressed is to get your body moving. Motion can change your emotion. Some examples could be putting on your yoga, dance, or Tai Chi DVD. You could also say to your child, "Shall we go for a walk? Or "Shall we go to the gym or leisure center?" Or "Why don't you call a friend and see if you can go kick a ball in the park." Do something physical! Exercise is a mood enhancer and stimulates the release of endorphins that we need to boost our sense of courage.

The second tip is to read something uplifting to keep you inspired and help you find the will to be courageous. Reading can be so important, both for you and your children. We are all interested in reading different kinds of things. Find a philosopher or a poet or a historian whose words can help you. Your children might be interested in something different than you. Sometimes children only like pictures or rhyming stories, but often they are attracted to the ideas. Notice what your child wants to read.

The essence of resiliency, and why it is such a vital resource, is this: resilience provides us with the existential courage that facilitates and drives our pursuit of finding purpose and meaning in our lives. Resiliency consolidates and catalyzes our energy and fortitude for confronting and surviving crises. But resiliency is much more than a resource to survive a crisis; it continues to assist us in making meaning of the crisis, gifting us with a vital perspective. It encourages us to not only learn from the crisis but finally to re-focus our energies on the future. And this is where emotional resiliency is critical.

Resilient individuals are characterized by not being satisfied with the status quo of the past. They are future-oriented decision-makers. For many, the future is perceived as holding too many unknowns and risks, creating anxiety and fear. A resilient person would rather work through the fear and anxiety of not knowing than experience the emotions associated with missed opportunities and the feelings of failure and guilt for not having the courage to pursue the future.

Emotional resiliency is about how we choose to use our emotions, and resilient individuals use their emotions as tools of insight in evaluating choices and the benefits of each choice. The key in resiliency is to facilitate emotional energy for transformational rather than regressive coping purposes. Our coping style is determined by our degree of tolerance for uncomfortable and unpleasant feelings. A resilient approach recognizes, acknowledges, and tolerates unpleasant emotions. And tolerating an emotion does not mean that you do nothing with the emotion. Instead, tolerating provides the space and opportunity to investigate the basis for the emotion and judge which response will benefit one's growth and full life.

Emotional Resiliency – For When The Going Gets Tough

There's nothing comfortable about conflict...but then where would we be without it? If you believe in Darwin's theory of natural selection, then you would relate to the fact that conflict is in our DNA as it is in all species. Without it, whose view would we adopt? Whose decisions would we accept? How would we react if things didn't work out as planned? Conflict is often seen as chaos because of our focus on the problem. However, conflict can also carry the opportunity to challenge current thinking, leverage creativity, and bring about change. But to achieve this, we must first embrace it with a mindset and focus on Outcomes (mutual needs) as opposed to Positional Thinking (self needs).

Our ability to move through conflict and change can certainly be defining moments for all of us. Consider for a moment, how do you respond when challenged? When people are nasty...do you switch off and wonder: "Why bother? This person doesn't deserve my help, let alone my respect....no way." Do you become emotionally compromised in the face of adversity, or do you exercise "emotional resilience" and accept what is happening and proactively seek to improve outcomes?

Experiencing unpleasant things is perhaps an important part of helping us to develop a deeper sense of appreciation for the more pleasant things. In contrast, relationships with people will have both good times and bad and smooth and rough periods. Situations will sometimes provide a reward, while at other times, they will be the opposite. Furthermore, not everything others do, want, or say at any given time is always going to suit our needs. Therefore we need to develop a sense of "hardiness" within ourselves to help us address these everyday challenges in life.

Without exercising emotional resilience, we might not have the capacity to work through the challenges of conflict or have the ability to endure differences. Moreover, we might not develop our capacity for patience and tolerance; after all, emotional challenges can get very uncomfortable. Rather we might seek solace in our need for "immediate gratification," which can take many forms, i.e., avoidance/withdrawal - walking away to evade dealing with the challenge or not engage in dialogue to prevent mediating difference, not take the time to see the value in another's an opinion, not seek to understand another's perspective, but rather get frustrated when things don't go our way or when people oppose us.

Embrace "Emotional Resilience" as a character trait to be admired, fostered, and developed. Communicating enables us to tolerate hardship without abandoning faith while continuing to pave the way forward for mutual benefit.

Emotional resilience provides us with a capacity to be more robust under stress conditions, particularly where we are personally challenged. It's an important life/work skill and worthy of us all considering and developing. And the good news is we all can, with a little focus and attention, **on two key "emotional intelligence competencies":**

- **Your sense of "Self Awareness"** – having a balanced and honest view of your personality and character traits, particularly under stress, and your ability to sense how emotions and behaviors affect both you and others.
- **Your capacity for "Self Control"** – your ability and willpower to control your emotions, particularly under stress and your thinking and behavior, especially in terms of your feelings and reactions towards impulses, desires, and wants.

Three key points to help you build "Emotional Resilience":

- Practice tolerating difficult behavior and opposing opinions, recognize that having your ideas, views, and values challenged is part of human behavior and life. Rather than focusing on the differences in positions, seek to value others' views, show respect and establish common ground upon which to build.
- Try to exercise patience by remaining receptive, open, and outcome-focused and seeking to improvise instead of getting bogged down. Focus more on proactively looking forwards and seeking mutual outcomes rather than looking back and apportioning blame or feeling like a victim.
- Focus on being respectful towards others in the way you communicate with them, through what you say, and the characteristics of your behavior. This is particularly the case when opinions differ from yours.

Mental Toughness And Resilience Helps Achieve Goals

Whatever system or method you prefer to use to choose and plan your goals, and there are many of them out there, once you've taken the vital first step forward, then you'll need mental toughness and resilience to keep going in the right direction.

Mental toughness as a concept is hard to define and pin down as it can mean many different things to many different people and in many different contexts.

In terms of achieving goals, mental toughness (MT) can be characterized by the ability to focus strongly on your outcome and the planned steps you need to take to achieve it. Sustained focus takes effort, and effort also requires mental toughness. There's a great deal of circularity involved.

A strong belief can also characterize mental toughness.

Believe that what you're striving for is of value to yourself and others.

Mental toughness can be further characterized by maintaining discipline for the task and avoiding distractions, which closely links with the need to focus.

There'll inevitably be various minor and major obstacles, setbacks, and failures along the way to your goal. Mental toughness is required to continually see beyond these and use their feedback to move forward. This also takes resilience.

The term resilience can best be described by using an analogy. Trees are things that we associate with strength and solidity. The secret to a tree being able to withstand hostile natural elements is an ability to bend with the wind and snow and then to bounce back when they're gone. The tree is flexible rather than rigid. The tree is resilient.

In moving forward toward achieving your goals, you'll need to be flexible and adaptable enough to learn from problems and knock-backs, and even from successes, and find alternative routes to your goal if necessary. This is true resilience.

Mental toughness and resilience are like the muscles in your body. In a similar way to muscles, they take training to grow and develop. They'll also atrophy and weaken with lack of use. They'll also tired with overuse, so give yourself some "you time" now and again to regroup and restore your energy. Keep developing these goal muscles, and with time and practice, you will find that achieving your goals becomes easier and more enjoyable.

Six Important Keys To Building Your Resilience Skills

Imagine you're going to take a raft trip down a river. Along with slow water and shallows, your map shows that you will encounter unavoidable rapids and turns. How would you make sure you can safely cross the rough waters and handle any unexpected problems from the challenge?

Resilience refers to how well you can deal with and bounce back from the difficulties of life. It can mean the difference between handling pressure and losing your cool. Resilient people tend to maintain a more positive outlook and cope with stress more effectively.

The good news is that even if you're not a naturally resilient person, you can learn to develop a resilient mindset and attitude. To do so, **incorporate the following into your daily life:**

- *Prioritize relationships.*

Connecting with empathetic and understanding people can remind you that you're not alone in the midst of difficulties. Focus on finding trustworthy and compassionate individuals who validate your feelings, which will support the skill of resilience.

The pain of traumatic events can lead some people to isolate themselves, but it's important to accept help and support from those who care about you. So whether you go on a weekly date night with your spouse or plan a lunch out with a friend, try to prioritize genuinely connecting with people who care about you.

- *Learn from your mistakes and failures.*

Every mistake has the power to teach you something important, so look for the lesson in every situation. Also, make sure that you understand the idea of "post-traumatic growth." Often, people find that crises, such as a job loss or the breakdown of a relationship, allow them to re-evaluate their lives and make positive changes.

- *Choose your response.*

Remember, we all experience bad days, and we all go through our share of crises. But we choose how we respond: we can choose to react with panic and negativity, or we can choose to remain calm and logical to find a solution. Your reaction is always up to you.

- *Maintain perspective.*

Resilient people understand that, although a situation or crisis may seem overwhelming at the moment, it may not make that much of an impact over the long term. Therefore, try to avoid blowing events out of proportion.

- *Set yourself some goals.*

If you don't already, learn to set SMART, effective personal goals that match your values, which can help you learn from your experiences.

- *Build your self-confidence.*

Remember, resilient people, are confident that they will succeed eventually, despite the setbacks or stresses they might face. This belief in themselves also enables them to take risks: when you develop confidence and a strong sense of self, you have the strength to keep moving forward and to take the risks you need to get ahead.

Getting help when you need it is crucial in building your resilience. The important thing is to remember you're not alone on the journey. While you may not control all of your circumstances, you can grow by focusing on the aspects of life's challenges you can manage with the support of loved ones and trusted professionals.

Five Secrets To Increase Resiliency In Yourself

Resiliency is the ability to bounce back when it seems like life strikes out at you – to take whatever comes your way, handle it, learn from it and continue. Resiliency comes into play when really difficult situations arise, such as relationship break up, death of a loved one, loss of career - in fact, any big financial challenge – helping someone you love (including yourself) with addiction, and so on.

But resiliency goes far beyond that - it also factors into your daily existence... whether it be continuing to go to a job you dislike day after day; forcing yourself to go for treatments at the doctor that you would rather not, or even bringing up a difficult conversation that could result in a confrontation with somebody that you're not ready for.

It is resiliency that stops a person from giving up on life completely, and it is resiliency that you use to pick yourself up and start piecing your life back together when you hit rock bottom.

So what can you do? **Here are the 5 tips to help you get started:**

- *Believe in your abilities.*

Having confidence in your ability to cope with the stresses of life can play an important part in resilience. Becoming more confident in your abilities, including your ability to respond to and deal with a crisis, is a great way to build resilience for the future.

Listen for negative comments in your head. Then, when you hear them, practice immediately replacing them with positive ones, such as, "I can do this," "I'm a great friend/mother/partner," or "I'm good at my job."

- *Embrace change.*

Flexibility is an essential part of resilience. By learning how to be more adaptable, you'll be better equipped to respond when faced with a life crisis. In addition, resilient people often utilize these events as an opportunity to branch out in new directions. While abrupt changes may crush some people, highly resilient individuals can adapt and thrive.

- *Be optimistic.*

Staying optimistic during dark periods can be difficult, but maintaining a hopeful outlook is an important part of resiliency. What you are dealing with may be difficult, but it's important to remain hopeful and positive about a brighter future.

Positive thinking does not mean ignoring the problem to focus on positive outcomes. Instead, it means understanding that setbacks are temporary and that you have the skills and abilities to combat the challenges you face.

- *Nurture yourself.*

When you're stressed, it can be all too easy to neglect your own needs. Losing your appetite, ignoring exercise, and not getting enough sleep are common reactions to a crisis situation. Instead, focus on building your self-nurturance skills, even when you're troubled. Make time for activities that you enjoy.

- *Take action.*

Simply waiting for a problem to go away on its own only prolongs the crisis. Instead, start working on resolving the issue immediately. While there may not be any fast or simple solution, you can take steps toward making your situation better and less stressful.

Focus on the progress you have made thus far and planning your next steps rather than becoming discouraged by the work that still needs to be accomplished.

So don't be afraid to think outside of the box or even use the box in a new and unexpected way. The more you do this, the more powerful you will feel.

CHAPTER 7

POSITIVE MENTAL ATTITUDE
– EXPLODING THE MYTH

There is something about everything that you can be glad about if you keep hunting long enough to find it.

Life certainly has its challenges, but it's a lot more satisfying when you choose to face the ups and downs with a smile. Continue reading to learn how to keep your chin up and why doing so matters in life.

A positive mental attitude sees the benefits, opportunities, and good in situations rather than the setbacks, problems, and bad. More important, it is focusing on this positive and using it to your advantage. PMA is asking how something can be done rather than saying it can't be done. It is the driving force behind persistence and perseverance.

A positive mental attitude. But what is attitude anyway? Simply put, it's the way you communicate your mood to others. In a deeper sense, it's the way you see the world or the way you choose to see the world. Because fortunately, having a positive attitude is a choice. Of course, no one can have a perfectly positive mental attitude all the time as things go wrong.

Sometimes your daily appointments get canceled, rejection

comes your way, and daily problems arise. Negative thoughts start to alter your perspective. Suppose you continually let the negative all-around takeover. In that case, you'll find yourself developing a chronically negative attitude, which weakens the spirit, produces energy, and saps enthusiasm for yourself and those around you.

Here's something to keep in mind, just as a cold or flu virus can be spread to others, so can Attitude. Studies have shown that mood is contagious. In one study, individuals in work teams began passing their moods to others within two hours. What's even more fascinating about this phenomenon known as emotional contagion is that leader's moods hold particular sway over their team members. So what does this mean to you as a leader or aspiring leader in your organization? You have tremendous power to influence the performance of your team. One of the most effective ways to successfully lead your organization is to be simply positive.

Tips for Staying Positive Throughout Your Life

You can do things to cultivate a positive mental attitude despite the challenges that will surely arise. **Here are some practical suggestions to help you and your team members look on the bright side of life, and find the strength to get up each time you fall.**

- **Be Grateful.** Gratitude is a virtue that helps you focus on the good things in life and see the bigger picture. When you concentrate on what matters most, your perspective widens from the tree in front of you until you see the whole forest. Even through rough times, there are many things you can be thankful for. Make it a daily habit to identify specific things you're grateful for doing. This will help you cultivate a positive attitude as you train your mind to focus on the good things in life.

- **Make Humor Part of Your Daily Life.** Laughter and a good sense of humor are key elements of a positive attitude. They reduce stress and anxiety. They strengthen relationships, and they elevate mood and hope. When you feel low, turn to comic strips of the funny sitcom, online jokes. Whatever makes you laugh. Look on the lighter side of things in your daily activities. Humor will help you keep a more optimistic view of life.

- **Inspiring Books.** Always keep a positive, inspiring book on hand when you're feeling down. Turn to a motivational passage, and give yourself a quick boost. Good books can inspire, encourage, and teach you. Also, reading requires you to stay still, and focusing on something uplifting will help you maintain a positive mental attitude.

- **Exercise.** Besides providing undeniable benefits to your physical health, exercise can also make a difference in mental health. Researchers have found that exercise combats stress and depression and improving mood and attitude. Also, don't overlook the connection between yourself looking good and feeling good. Imagine a positive attitude when you feel and look physically; you gain confidence and see things with more bright eyes.

- **Give Service.** There's something magical about helping others in need. It causes you to forget your problems and your motive becomes their wellness. Right around the next time you're stuck in an "all about me" mindset, put this principle to the test. You'll find there's great euphoria in doing something to bless the life of another without any thought or expectation of a reward.

- **Surround Yourself With Positive People.** Negativity is even more contagious than the common cold. It spreads like a wildfire that is out of control, and the best way to avoid it is to stay out of its path.

The power of a positive mental attitude each day brings new challenges that demand the best of you, and the way you choose to base that will determine much of your growth. Success and happiness, cultivating the gift of a positive attitude, will change your perspective and help you see your goals more clearly. You'll surely make life more enjoyable. Could you do it for yourself and those around you? Remember, it's your choice to choose to look on the bright side!

Why Emotional Resilience Means Handling Ambiguity Fluidly

Resilience means living well with ambiguity; of having learned to live with conflicting ideas. Resilience, in this way, can refer to our tolerance for the wavering extremes of situational experience - the steadier we are emotional, the more resilient we are.

This is what Paul meant when he said, "I have learned to be content with whatever I have." (Philippians 4:11)

Paul must have meant that he could deal with both blessed and cursed situations - that neither could dissuade him from the stable foundational underpinnings of his faith. Pride would not be a problem when things were going well. And despair would not be a problem when things were not going so well.

Nobody truly puts themselves in harm's way and claims a certain portion of wisdom unless they do so selflessly for others. Likewise, those with emotional resilience will not willingly put themselves on the frontline without reason, but if God calls them to represent a good cause, they will front up and fight the good fight.

As a person deals patiently with stress and ambiguity, bearing both consternation and confusion gallantly, they show great emotional resilience.

It isn't until we are tested that we know the true make-up of our character. And the truth is many times; we will fail the tests that are brought our way. Fortunately, God provides us many second chances to exemplify resilience.

We cannot judge the resilience of a person until they have suffered. It is no blessing to anyone to have avoided suffering. It is the putting off of the inevitable. Inevitably we will all suffer, and it is only through the bearing of that suffering that we are to grow in resilience because of the compassion nurtured within.

Emotional resilience is the compensation of God for the suffering we have entered into with an attitude aligned to God's will. God does not will for us to suffer, but he does will our stately response. When we respond faithfully to God's faithfulness to see us right, we stand out of the way of cursing, and we allow God to bless us because we have stood out of the way of cursing the injustice.

Emotional resilience doesn't come to the fore until a genuine test comes. It's a break-glass-in-an-emergency faculty. We know we are made of the right stuff when we do the right stuff in the time of trouble. Resilience, therefore, was made for the storm, and only in a storm does it vindicate us.

Resilience Does Not Begin With Strategies - It Begins With YOU

Resilience is one of the essential soft leadership skills for changing and challenging times. Leaders and managers need to be constantly developing the resilience of their people. Here are the seven most important qualities people need to develop if they want to bounce back from adversity in these turbulent times:

- *Develop self-awareness- so you know what's stopping you from being resilient.*

The more we know and understand ourselves, the more empowered we feel. When we become aware of what makes us tick, what challenges and threatens us or heightens our anxiety, what creates overwhelm and stress, what keeps us awake at night, we can then take charge of it, rather than it taking charge of us. We don't get stuck. We break through our stuff and move forward quickly. We are resilient.

Key question: What major aspect of your personality or life needs most work to be resilient?

- *Develop a positive explanatory style.*

We all have an explanatory style - a way we explain to ourselves why things happen. We can have a negative style where we see life as a conspiracy, out to get us, disempowers us, and makes us feel helpless. We can have a positive style that always sees a way forward that empowers and encourages proactivity. Only people with a positive explanatory style will be resilient.

Key question: How do you explain to yourself and those close to you why setbacks happen in your life?

- *Become proactive.*

Resilience is a very dynamic and action-oriented quality. It involves a response from the whole self - body, heart, mind, and spirit. People who stay in challenging situations resign themselves to them and manage by disengaging and switching off because they feel powerless and helpless to do anything about it are not resilient people. To be resilient, they need to take a proactive response.

Key question: How long does it take you, when something goes wrong in your life or work, to assume a proactive position that will turn it around - an hour, day, week, more than a week?

- *Be a problem solver.*

Be someone who focuses on solutions, not problems, but be reflective enough to ask new questions that might generate new answers, not time-honored solutions. Be constructive, strategic, analytical, goal focussed.

Key question: What qualities do you bring to problem-solving situations?

- *Develop emotional maturity and intelligence.*

Be aware of your emotional responses to situations and experiences - fear, guilt, anxiety, depression, anger, and frustration. Bring both your head and heart to those emotions so that your responses are informed by good, balanced judgment. Learn to exist creatively in tension and how to grow through pain. Resilient people do not suppress emotion; they take hold of it and drive them to solutions.

Key question: What are the emotions that obstruct you from taking action and moving forward after adversity?

- *Look after yourself.*

Alcohol, drugs, junk food, sugar fixes, cigarettes, sleeping tablets, and caffeine do not produce resilient people. Healthy, natural, unprocessed food, exercise, water, time to smell the roses, sleep, meditation, contemplation, and reflection give people the energy, clear-headedness, and focus they need to be resilient.

Key question: How can you look after yourself and prime your body, heart, and mind so that you can proactively respond to whatever challenges present themselves to you?

- *Embracing change.*

Change is one of the only certainties in life. It brings with it unpredictability, confusion, uncertainty, paradox, and ambiguity. It can shake our foundations and challenge our value systems, leaving us feeling insecure and vulnerable. Resisting change heightens its impact. Working with change, rather than being threatened by it, is what resilient people do.

Key question: What is it about change that is threatening to you?

Many of you reading this will probably feel that these 7 developmental actions are not specific enough for you to do anything about. Developing resilience is about developing inner strength and toughness. The changes we need to make within ourselves are indeed difficult to make by ourselves.

Empath Yoga: A New Approach To Emotional Resiliency

Perhaps the biggest challenge in today's world is to experience all
of life - the joy, ecstasy, and bliss, along with the disappointment,
heartbreak, and pain, and still keep an open heart - to remain
fully awake, aware, and alive. But without this conscious intention,
many of us will shut down, become guarded, reactive and
defensive. Yoga is a powerful tool to help us release tension in the
body, quiet the mind, and soften and open the heart.

We've all been hurt before and experienced disappointment,
heartbreak, and loss. Without knowing how important it is to let
this energy move through us, we begin to let past hurts dictate our
future rather than shutting down around it. Physically this shows
up with a slouched posture and rounded shoulders as we collapse
in on ourselves in an attempt to protect our hearts from future
wounds.

From the earliest age, most of us have been receiving messages
that it is not okay to feel anger, sadness, insecurity, fear, or any
other emotion that is deemed negative. For many, this showed up
in statements like "stop crying or I'll give you a reason to cry" or
"boys don't cry," or even "stop being so emotional." With these
words and others, we were taught that anything other than
happiness and joy is not valid, and so begins the guilt and shame
surrounding so many of our lives.

Now, as adults, and after a lifetime of stuffing our emotions
deep inside, many of us are brimming over with that which has
remained undealt with. Yet it still keeps calling to us, stalking our
every move and nipping at our heels, waiting for us to stop long
enough to allow all that we have been running from to catch up
with us.

This isn't the only compulsive behavior we engage in, which is
why over 64% of Americans are overweight or obese. Even with

these coping mechanisms, insomnia affects more than half of the U.S. population, with as many as 58% of adults complaining of sleepless nights at least a few times a week.

But perhaps the most alarming statistic of all is that anti-depressant usage is up 800% in the last 10 years. This trend toward disowning what's coming up inside is affecting us at younger and younger ages, and sadly it is pre-schoolers that are the fastest-growing market.

All of this points to the fact that it's time for us to stop running away from ourselves. True emotional resiliency means giving ourselves enough credit to know we can allow ourselves to feel what we need to feel, confident that once we do and come out on the other side of it, we will be lighter, and stronger, and more at ease than ever before, perhaps since we were children.

There has developed such a disconnection between our minds and our bodies, many of us have become lost in an endless stream of mental chatter that is so busy, we have become like heads walking around without bodies. We become so lost in the thoughts, the story, the illusion that we no longer have a relationship with or even feel our bodies. Yet, it connects us to what is happening inside our bodies that connect us to our center and grounds us.

Most of us believe we are healthy enough to spend time and energy focusing on caring for our physical bodies and intellectual pursuits. But very little attention is being paid to our emotional wellness, which is the same energy that fuels us, and it affects the quality of our lives. For many, long after they have cared for the needs of their physical body and stimulated their minds with intellectual pursuits, emotional health is the last frontier.

But this is a beautiful time we are living in. As the world around us changes rapidly, more and more people are turning their focus inward. When the world outside appears crazy, it's the only place left to go.

And no journey of self-discovery can go far without a willingness to recognize what it is we are feeling. Something as subtle as a feeling can be easily ignored in a world with so much mental noise and external distraction vying for our attention. But without a willingness to see, own and understand the subtle energy that moves through our bodies, we can never truly know ourselves.

Our feelings always have a message for us. And if we choose to ignore them, our body starts sending louder, clearer messages that will eventually manifest as dis-ease in the body if denied long enough. Denying our feelings is like holding a beach ball underwater; it cannot be held down forever and eventually will push its way to the surface.

All too often, we wait until we are on our knees, exhausted from trying to impose our will on a situation unsuccessfully before we are humbled enough to stop, pay attention, and start opening our minds to the possibility of a new way.

This is what inspired the birth of Empath Yoga, a yoga immersion experience and certification course. Empath Yoga is the natural culmination of nearly a decade of work and experience with individuals and groups worldwide. The approach is simple: provide a safe place for clients to get in touch with their truth, to feel what they need to feel so they can come out on the other side of it, and support and empower them to make powerful choices in their lives.

The sense of lightness of being that comes from letting go - of the tension we unknowingly hold onto in our bodies, of the restricting old tapes that we replay in our minds, and of the feelings that we have stuffed deep inside - is unlike anything that can be described in words. It must be felt. It must be experienced.

Resilience: A Key To A Successful Today And Tomorrow

Success in business and life comes to those who can sustain energy, creativity, and passion in the midst of continual change, stress, and competition. Information overload leaves us struggling to sustain that passion and drive and achieve the work/life balance essential to our growth and well-being. We are being bombarded with information every day and are working in different environments that require more accountability and have higher expectations than 10 years ago.

Individual and organizational resilience is needed now more than ever. Webster's Dictionary defines resilience as the ability to recover from misfortune or change. It is also defined as the integrated power to persist when things don't work out at first, navigate ambiguity and uncertainty, transcend common problems and barriers, and sustainably anticipate the future.

Individuals are instilled with certain capabilities that define what it is like to be human. Among those capabilities are: the ability to learn from our mistakes, plan for the future, reflect on ourselves and situations and manage our emotions. These capabilities provide us with the tools to control our future and remain resilient in changing times. Developing these capabilities is the key to increasing our resilience. They are what make us human. We are the only species that is capable of planning, reflecting, and managing our emotions. So the elements that make us unique are the same elements that can make us resilient in challenging times.

Resilience matters more than training, education, and experience and will ultimately determine who succeeds and fails.

There are many elements of resilience, but these are the ones I find most important:

- **Accept things as they are, not as you hope or wish they would be.** It is easy to slip into denial to cope with challenging times, but the only real way to prepare ourselves and our organizations for these challenges is to face reality. When we deny things, we perpetuate the hardship and stop any growth and renewal from occurring. With each day and month, the cost of denial goes up. To be truly resilient, an individual and an organization must avoid wishful thinking and stop living in the past. They must be willing to face reality head-on. Resilience means having the capacity to change before the change becomes necessary. This is planning for our futures rather than being victims of our reality.

- **Know what's important and navigate around that.** When there is a lack of clarity around what is most important, our actions and behaviors are undirected, and resilience is stalled. Strong values serve as maps to guide our behaviors and actions. At times of crisis and hardships, this clarity allows us to navigate through the fog. If we are lost with no map and no signs to guide us, it makes recovery much longer. Successful individuals and organizations have strong values that direct their behavior at times of crisis.

- **Know Thy Self.** Self Knowledge is critical for resilience. If we are clear about our strengths and weaknesses, we can better leverage our strengths and manage our weaknesses. When we spend much of our time operating out of our weaknesses, more effort is expended, and results are dispersed. Directing our actions around our strengths allows us to be more efficient and effective in freeing up creative energy.

Problems and challenges will not be transcended if we become victims of our blind spots and minimize our talents and creativity.

- **Accept and make meaning out of what life hands us.** The core of resilience is the ability to bounce back from hardships. If we complain and whine about the challenges upon us, we cannot adequately reflect and learn from the difficulties. Resilient people and organizations can see a potential opportunity hidden beneath adversity. They build bridges with reflections from their past to the ingenuity of today and finally to a fuller future.

The resilient people of today and tomorrow are the ones who can face reality head-on, knowing what's important at the moment, leveraging their strengths, and making meaning out of hardships. We create the future through our response to the challenges of today.

CONCLUSION

Mental immunity is bolstered hugely by your nervous system spending time in its resting (or "parasympathetic") state. Sleep is good; however, telling anyone with sleep problems to sleep more is just cruel. Instead, make time for active rest – take a long bath, read a book (with your phone off), do a puzzle, or try deep belly breathing or yin yoga.

While it's tempting to push difficult or painful emotions aside, doing so just creates more space for them to thrive. If you're feeling anxious, sad, lonely, confused, or anything else, you are by no means alone. Acknowledge these feelings to yourself and your loved ones, and give yourself the space to process them so that they don't weigh you down. If it helps – scream, cry, shout, hit a pillow – do what you need to get your emotions out.

Exercise is proven to almost always help improve your mood – both in the short and long term. If you're feeling terrible, it's very hard to do anything at all, so it's helpful to start a regular movement habit when you're feeling okay and then keep reminding yourself of the power of endorphins when you're not. It doesn't matter how you move – walk, dance, box, stretch – just pick something that works for you.

The more you associate yourself with your mental health difficulties, the harder it becomes to separate them.

So if you are feeling depressed or anxious, remind yourself that that doesn't make you an anxious or depressed person – it just means that that's what you're experiencing right now. Things are always in flux, and you are much more than the sum of your current state of mind.